# THE WELLPRENEUR PLANNER

A YEAR OF INCREDIBLE GROWTH FOR YOUR WELLNESS BUSINESS

# THE WELLPRENEUR PLANNER

A YEAR OF INCREDIBLE GROWTH FOR YOUR WELLNESS BUSINESS

Amanda Cook

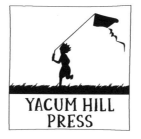

Published by Yacum Hill Press

Wellpreneur is a registered trademark of Wellpreneur Ltd.

To purchase multiple copies, or for interviews with Amanda, please contact info@amandacook.me or visit her website: https://AmandaCook.me

ISBN: 978-0-9957443-2-5

Editing: Gillian Katsoulis
Book Design: Chiara Pennella
Author Photo: Melissa Grapp

WELLPRENEUR (N):

*An entrepreneur in the field of health and wellness.*
*An entrepreneur who considers and prioritizes personal and communal well being while building a business.*

# Table of Contents

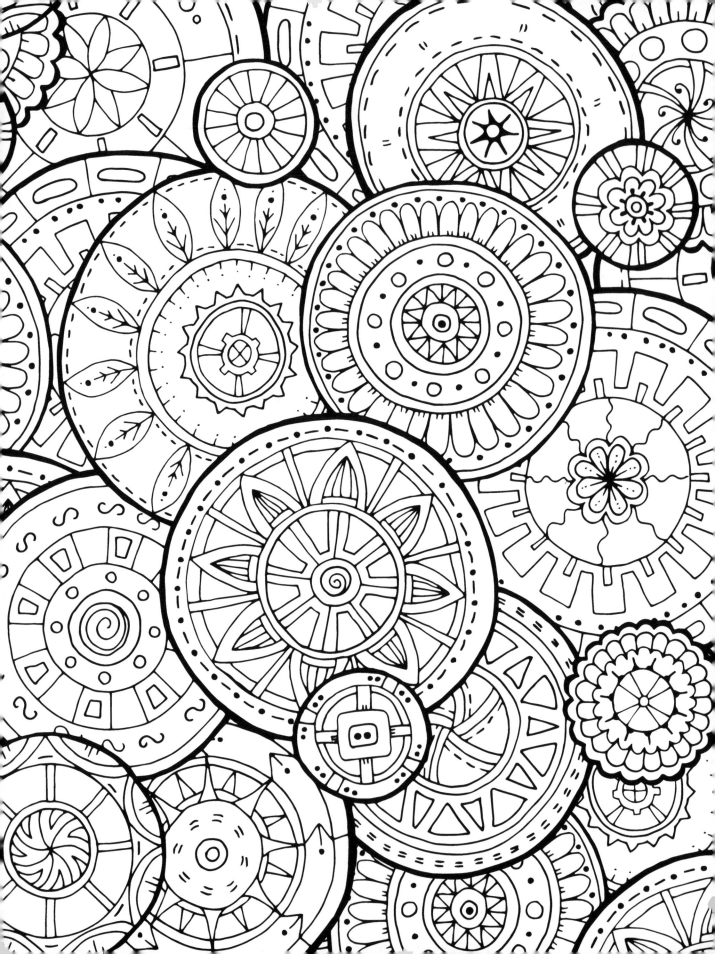

# How to Use This Planner

- This is a 12-month planner that can start any time. No need to wait for January! You'll plan the next year starting from today.
- Start the planner when you're in a positive, creative, growth-oriented mood. You might meditate, do a gratitude practice, exercise, or listen to your favorite music to prime yourself to dream big.
- Grab a cup of tea, coffee or wine — but not too much! You want to be relaxed and creative, not tipsy, foggy or jittery!
- Use a good pen (so your writing, dreaming and doodling flows...).
- Go to a place where you can focus. The best location may not be your daily workspace. Going to a fresh location can spark creative ideas.
- Don't worry about having the "right" answers. Just complete the planner from where you are right now. If a section does not apply to you, just skip it and move forward.
- I give you permission to be creative in planning your year. Write, doodle, color in the pictures, flag pages with sticky notes — it's your planner, make it work for you.
- Consider finding an accountability buddy. Complete your planners separately, then get together (in person or virtually) to review your dreams, plans and action steps.
- And finally, keep this planner somewhere you can review it regularly. It's designed to be an integral part of your year, keeping you on track to bring your big vision to life — and to track your progress along the way.

# Welcome, Wellpreneur!

In your hands, you have the ultimate planner and workbook to create the best year yet for your wellness business!

This planner contains a powerful process to shift from dreaming to doing, attract your tribe of ideal clients and create a thriving wellness business through authentic online marketing.

Over the past six years of working with wellness entrepreneurs at various stages of business (plus having used numerous strategies on my own natural health and beauty blog), I've seen what separates those who get clients from those who don't.

*Clarity + Focus = Results*

There are hundreds of ways to bring clients to your wellness business, but you can't do them all. You have to choose. Success comes from setting out a clear path to get in front of the right people, build relationships, and make offers — and then sticking with it! That's the process I'll guide you through in this planner.

Because you're a wellpreneur, I'm guessing you're passionate about health and wellness. Your business isn't simply a path to wealth, it's the next phase in your life's work. That's why it's extra-important that you stay focused on your big vision, so you know WHY you're doing this work and aren't distracted by the latest shiny marketing tactic!

Here's how the planner works:

We'll start by reviewing your previous 12 months. It doesn't matter if you're starting the planner in January, December or June — just look back at the last 12 months. If you're using this planner for a new business, still complete the previous 12 months, but from the perspective of your life/work/education (whichever is relevant). Not all question may apply to you, but there is still much wisdom you can glean from your personal experiences over the past year and we want to capture this wisdom to help plan your next year.

Next, we'll turn our focus towards what you're going to create in the next 12 months. You'll clarify your big dreams, dig deep into marketing to turn those dreams into reality, and identify where you need support along the way. We'll also look at bringing balance, ease and fun into your life so you can really make these plans happen. After all, what's the point of running your own wellness business if you're stressed out and overworked?

Finally, the planner closes with pages for planning and tracking progress each month. You'll be able to plan each month on a calendar, note your wins and lessons learned, and track your growth throughout the year!

I designed this planner as a companion to my book *Wellpreneur*, which teaches my Organic Growth System to bring more of the right people to your website and turn them into paying clients. The planner can be used on its own, but if you want a more in-depth explanation of setting up your online marketing (choosing a niche, creating an opt-in gift, blogging, newsletters, etc.), it's all in *Wellpreneur*.

My intention for this planner is that it is an active part of your business. It's meant to be used, not kept on a shelf: write, color, plan, doodle, add notes, track results — make it yours! Schedule monthly dates with yourself to track your progress, reconnect with your dreams and adjust your plans. It can go on the shelf at the end of the year as a record of how far you've come.

Dream big and keep going!

*Amanda*

Founder, Wellpreneur Ltd.
Host of The Wellpreneur Podcast

///////////
PS: You're not alone in planning an amazing year! Snap a pic of you working on your planner and share it with the hashtag #wellpreneurplanner

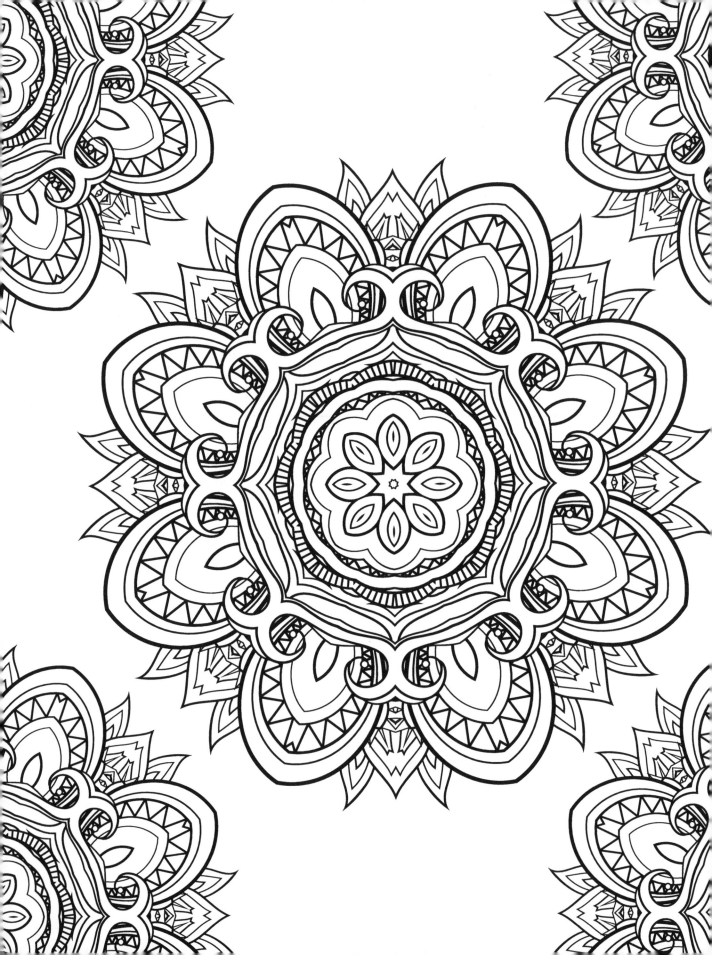

# LAST
# YEAR
___

Let's start crafting your amazing year by looking back at the reality of the past 12 months. We'll look at what worked and what didn't, your victories and failures, and most of all, the lessons you'll bring into the next year.

It doesn't matter whether the year was incredible or didn't unfold quite as you'd hoped. Don't judge, just observe what actually happened and capture it below. If you're starting a new business, answer these questions about your previous 12 months of life/work/education. Often, the challenges you experience at work or school will appear again in your own business.

You've probably noticed that we encounter the same lessons over and over until we integrate their teachings into our lives, so don't be modest about your victories or candy-coat your challenges. Good and bad, it's all valuable.

What were your life and business like one year ago today?

Did you have goals for the past year? What were they?

For each goal, what did you learn from the process of achieving it (or not)?

What was the goodness in the previous 12 months?
List 5 victories (big or small) that you're grateful for.

1. _____
2. _____
3. _____
4. _____
5. _____

What worked well?

What didn't work very well?

What did you LOVE about your business in the past year?

What did you really not enjoy? What could have been better?

Who supported you in your life and business?

# Your Word

I have an annual practice of choosing a word (you might think of it as a *theme*) to guide my year. If you also had a word or theme for last year, complete this section. If not, just skip to the next section — and don't worry, you'll have a word for next year (we'll get to that soon)!

### What was your word for the last year?

### How did you embody that word or theme?

Did you do anything to resist (or push back on) your word this year? If so, how?

What have you learned about yourself from this word?

# Know Your Numbers

It's easy to get caught up in the daily running of your business, and forget to look at the big picture growth. In this section, you'll capture metrics as they are today - and compare them to last year's numbers (if you know them.) If you don't know last year's numbers, just leave that column blank. Open your website dashboard, email marketing software and social media platforms. Do not skip this step! You'll thank me next year.

| YOUR EMAIL LIST | 1 YEAR AGO | TODAY |
|---|---|---|
| Number of email subscribers | | |
| Average email open rate | | |
| Average email click-through rate | | |

| SOCIAL MEDIA FOLLOWERS | 1 YEAR AGO | TODAY |
|---|---|---|
| Facebook page | | |
| Facebook group | | |
| Pinterest | | |
| Instagram | | |
| Twitter | | |
| YouTube | | |

| WEBSITE | 1 YEAR AGO | TODAY |
|---|---|---|
| Number of website visits per day or month | | |
| Most popular blog post or piece of content | | |
| Best-selling product or service | | |
| Revenue for the past 12 months | | |

| ANY OTHER METRICS RELEVANT TO YOUR BUSINESS | 1 YEAR AGO | TODAY |
|---|---|---|
| | | |
| | | |
| | | |
| | | |
| | | |
| | | |

# The Shape of Your Year

Now let's do a quick check on the overall shape of your year. You might think of this as work/life balance, but that's a slightly misleading term. There's no such thing as a "perfect" balance — it's unique for every person and it shifts throughout your life. Let's see what it looks like for you now.

Each line on the wheel indicates an element of your life. Feel free to adjust the labels to fit what you do and how you spend your time.

Draw a dot on each line indicating how satisfied you were with that area of your life in the past 12 months. A dot towards the center of the circle means "not satisfied at all," while a dot towards the edge of the wheel means "yes, totally satisfied!"

Once you have a dot on each line, connect each dot to the one next to it with a straight line. You'll finish with a shape that probably looks like a bumpy circle!

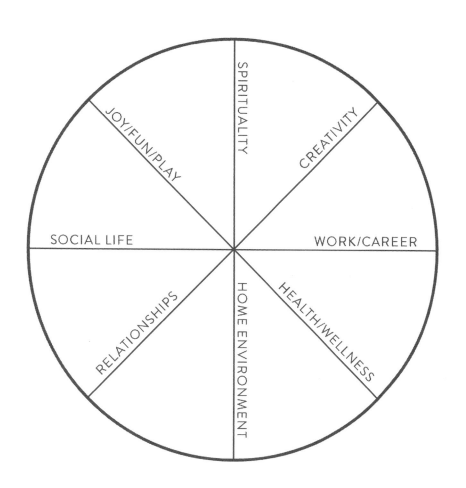

Which area are you most satisfied with?

What have you done this year to allow this area to flourish?

Which area would you most like to improve next year? *(Note: this isn't always the lowest area — it's the one which bothers you the most and that you actively want to improve.)*

What are three micro-actions you could take to improve this area?
*(A micro-action is an extremely small step which moves you in your desired direction.*
*A great micro-action should be quick and easy to do, in only one step.*
*Break any bigger tasks down into a series of micro-actions.)*

# The Wisdom of Last Year

Every lesson, no matter how painful, has a positive side and a shadow. Let's see what goodness we can take from all of the lessons this year.

### What wisdom will you take away from the last year?

### What have you learned about your business?

What have you learned about yourself?

What have you learned about what motivates you?

What truths have you uncovered?

# Closing the Year with Gratitude

Now, let's say THANK YOU to the year and send it off with gratitude. Write a few sentences of gratitude and appreciation to the past year as a way to bring closure.

/////////////

//////////////

At this point, you might choose to do a little closing ritual. You might write a thank you to the previous year on a piece of paper and burn it, or meditate, or do whatever else feels right to you. You might choose to take a little break from the planner and get outside into the sunshine, feeling a sense of closure and new beginnings. Or, you might just want to plunge ahead into dreaming big about the coming year and continue on with the planner. Go with what feels right to you, at this moment...

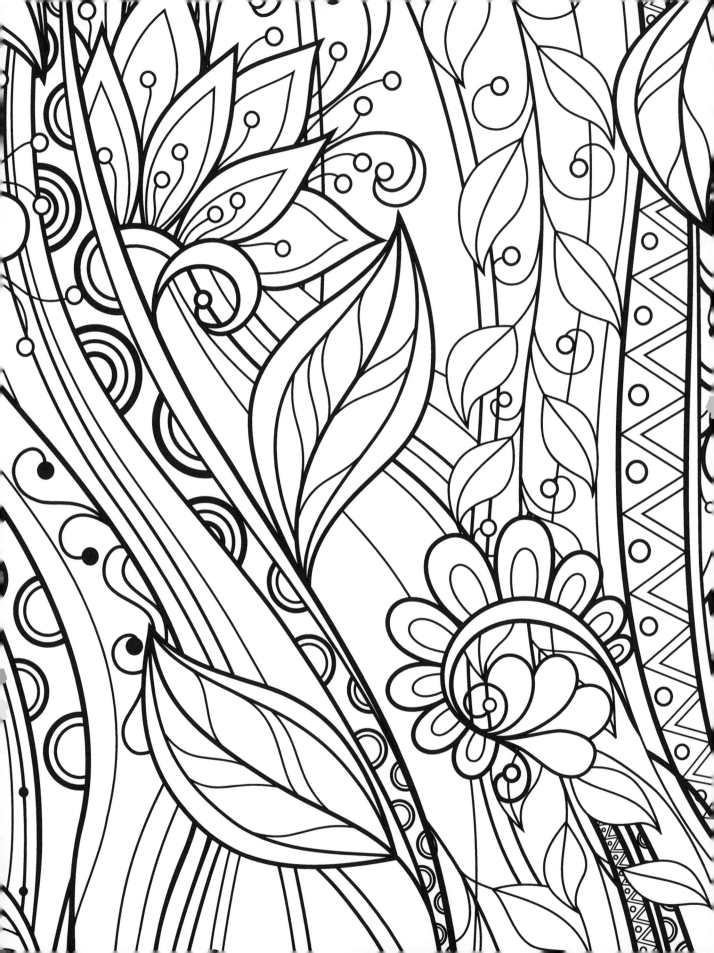

# THE YEAR AHEAD

# Your Big Dreams

Now let's turn our attention to the next 12 months. A year full of potential, growth, nourishment and stepping more fully into being YOU in every area of your life and business.

An incredible year starts with your big vision and dreams. After all, if you don't know where you're going, any road can get you there (thank you, Cheshire Cat!).

Many wellpreneurs avoid creating a clear life and business vision. This is partly out of fear: why risk imagining something that feels so good, if it might not become a reality? These fears are real, but they're not going to stop you this year.

In this planner, you're going to dream big — and then you'll break it down into the practical steps to get there. Trust that when you start taking steps in the right direction you'll experience opportunities you never imagined. But it's up to you to take those first brave steps into the unknown. Ready?

## PART 1: DREAMING

I want you to spend a little time *feeling into* what you want for your business and life. (Notice I said *feeling*, not *thinking*. Of course you'll use your brain, but let your heart and gut lead you in this section, not your intellectual mind!)

Close your eyes and imagine that you've done it. You've created your ultimate life and business. Savor that feeling. Let's join "future you" for a day in your ideal life.

Good morning! See yourself waking up.
• Where are you? Where do you live?
• Who is with you? What's your morning routine like?
• Do you go to work? Where?
• Are you alone or with others? What kind of tasks do you do during the day?
• What kind of clients or customers do you work with?
• What do you do in the afternoon? What about the evening?
• What are the most exciting things happening in your life and business that week, month or year?
• How do you feel about your life and business?
• What are you looking forward to in the future?

You might not know all the specific details, but just do the best you can. And most importantly, pay attention to the *feelings* you want to create. You might be surprised at what comes up.

## PART 2: FREE-WRITING

Now you're going to free-write about the dream life and business you just experienced. Silence the critical voice in your head that whispers "you can't do that!" "that's impossible," "how are you going to do that?" Don't worry about those doubts. **This is the time to get it all out on paper, not to figure out how you're going to do it. The "how" comes later.** For now, just write everything down.

Set a timer for 10 minutes and just allow your creativity and dreams to flow as you write about your ideal life. What would you like to create in your life and business? How do you want to feel? What do you dream about **doing, being and having?**

Make sure to specifically answer these questions:
- Where are you working?
- How do you work with your clients, customers or patients?
- Do you work: online, offline, or a mix of both?
- How much are you interacting with clients, customers or patients? 1:1? In groups? Not at all?
- Do you have a team, colleagues, coworkers?
- What other work activities do you do? Writing books? Speaking? Retreats? Workshops? Online courses? A podcast? TV appearances? What would make up your ultimate work life?

Don't let yourself get stuck here. You don't need to figure out exactly what your business and life are going to look like (after all, that's pretty much impossible). **What you want is to identify how you want to feel and the values that will influence your life and business.** There are no right or wrong answers — you can change and evolve this vision over time. Just be as specific as possible about what you want right now.

## PART 3: GETTING SPECIFIC

Looking back over your ideal life and business from the last activity, do the following:

List 5-7 words describing how you want to FEEL everyday:

What are some of the foundations that need to be in place to realize your dream life and business? For example, if you want to be a published author, you need to write a book. If you want to be location independent, you need to start creating products and services that don't require you to be in one place. List 3-5 foundational items here:

Now, for each foundational item, list 3-5 micro-actions that would take you in that direction:

# WORD OF THE YEAR

I love, love, love choosing a word of the year.

I touched on this briefly in the "Last Year" section, but now it's time to figure out the word that will guide you through the next year. Your word embodies what you want to be, do and have in the next 12 months. It's a simple but powerful practice that quickly brings you back into alignment with your goals and big picture dreams.

When trying to come up with a word for the year, it might pop into your head immediately — or you might need to play with it for awhile. If it's not immediate for you, brainstorm 10 or 20 different words until one 'clicks' and feels right. Consider what you want your focus to be — is it your business, your personal life, something else? What part of that do you want to improve or increase? You might find it helpful to review what you've written about your past 12 months as well as the feelings and ideas about your future.

Don't stress about this exercise, just let yourself choose the word that feels best. If you feel like you've "outgrown" the word before the end of the year, that's fine, you can pick a new one then.

You can use the space on the next page to brainstorm your word for the year. When you choose one, write it here.

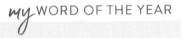
*my* WORD OF THE YEAR

BRAINSTORM YOUR IDEAS HERE

## OPTIONAL: CREATE A VISION BOARD

A vision board is a tool to quickly realign yourself with your ideal life and business. It's a collection of images and words that represent what you want to be, do, have and feel. It sounds woo woo, but in my experience, it really works!

Between you and me, I don't believe that simply choosing pictures of what you want magically makes them appear. I think vision boards work because they keep your big dreams and goals in the front of your mind, rather than lost in mental clutter and to-do lists. Fortunately, we don't need to know how they work to get value from the process. Here's how to make one.

**Make Your Vision Board**

- Do the visualizing and free-writing exercises earlier in this section to identify your big goals and dreams, and key words and concepts.
- Your vision board can be physical (a collage on paper or a bulletin board), or digital (a collage saved as an image on your computer).
- Choose the background for your vision board (a thick sheet of paper, bulletin board, or a blank page in your graphic design program).
- Play with images. Flip through magazines or scroll through Pinterest and cut out or save images which represent what you want to be, do, have and feel. I like to tear out images so they have rough, natural edges instead of sharp cuts — it's up to you!
- Glue (or place) them onto your board however appeals to you. Some people make a layered collage, others prefer straight edges.
- Finish by adding some words clipped from magazines, drawn, written, painted or typed onto your board.

Now the most important step — hang your vision board where you can see it easily. If you want the vision board technique to work for you, make it EASY. Where can you put your vision board so that you see it several times a day? In your office? Or what about in your kitchen or beside your bed?

You could set a digital vision board as your computer background or mobile phone screensaver. Any time you feel overwhelmed or lost or caught up in the details of running your business, just take a deep breath to center yourself and look at your vision board for a few seconds to reconnect with where you're going.

////////////

Share a picture of your vision board with the hashtag #wellpreneurplanner.

## KEEPING YOUR BIG VISION ALIVE...

It's so easy to get caught up in the day to day of life and business and lose sight of WHY you're doing this work. So, as we bring this dreaming section to a close, let's play with ways you can stay actively engaged with your big vision.

- Meditation
- Affirmations
- Journaling
- Sharing your vision with trusted friends/mastermind buddies
- Vision board
- Energy work
- Visualization

### How will you stay connected to your big vision?

///////////

Now with your big vision in mind, let's look at how you're
going to create it in the next 12 months...

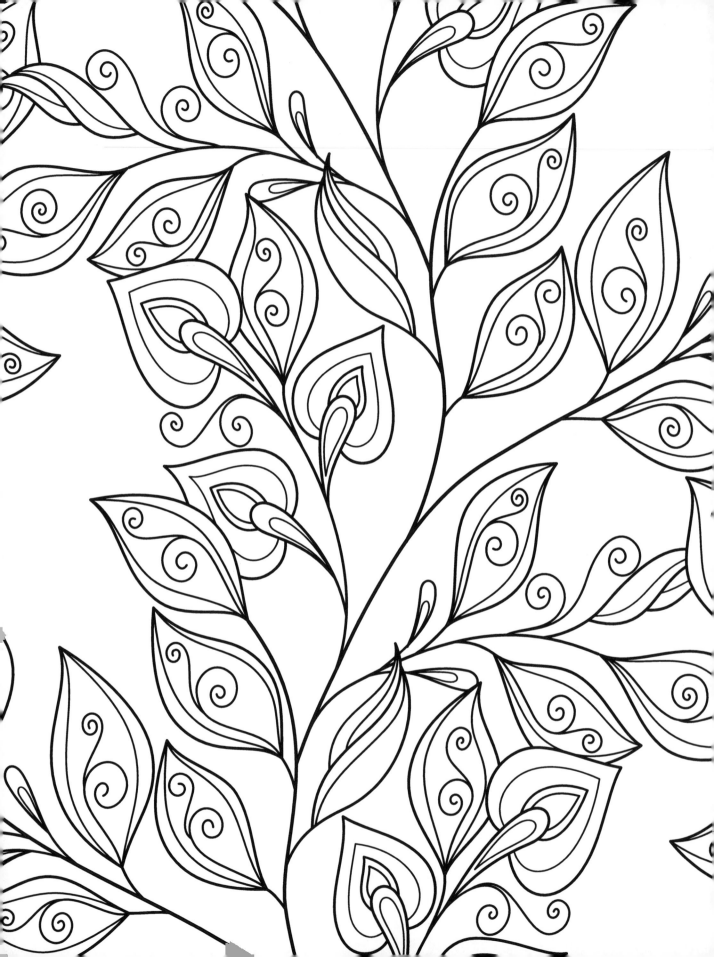

# FROM
# DREAMING
# TO DOING

———

Now that you're clear on your big vision for the next year, it's time to identify the concrete steps to make it happen. Here's how the rest of the planner works: We'll start by looking at the online marketing for your business. You'll see how to attract the right people to your business and how to turn them into paying clients. Then we'll dig into each step of this process in more detail, noting action steps along the way and incorporating your goals and dreams from the previous section. We'll then take this big list of actions and prioritize it, so you know where to start. Then we'll lay out the tasks month by month. The planner also includes a detailed section for each month to do more specific weekly planning and track your progress, wins and results!

Ready? Let's start with your online marketing.

When growing your wellness business using online marketing, you'll want to consistently increase your audience, develop your relationship with them, and then make relevant offers for your products and services.

It's important to see the big picture of how your business will grow online. A key part of this is understanding the exact path your clients follow from their initial interaction to becoming a paying client. I call this flow the Organic Growth System. Let's look at how the system works before we apply it to your business. (If you want more explanation, I cover this system and how to set it up in more depth in *Wellpreneur*.)

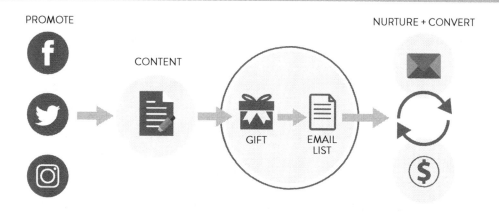

WELLPRENEUR ORGANIC GROWTH SYSTEM

PROMOTE

CONTENT

GIFT    EMAIL LIST

NURTURE + CONVERT

You might think you need to start with growing your social media following. In my experience, the best place to start is with your email list, because it's the core of your business. Here's why:

**The Core System: Your Email List and Opt-In Offer**

The core of your online wellness business is your email list. Having an email list gives YOU the power to contact your audience. Rather than hoping people will return to your website, having an email list means you can proactively contact your potential clients when you have something interesting to share or a new offer. The way you get people to join your email list is with a valuable free offer. Your free offer could be an ebook, mini course, video series, guided meditation, toolkit, coupon, or any other offer your potential followers might want. The key is that it has to actually be valuable for your ideal customer.

Your email list and opt-in offer are key to building your audience. But how will people find out about your opt-in offer?

**Your Valuable Free Content**

Content can take many forms based on your strengths and interests. The most common are writing (blogging), online video and audio (podcasts). Potential customers find your content, and then somewhere around that content (either at the end of the content or nearby on your website) they see your free offer. If they like your content and find it valuable, there's a good chance they'll take you up on your free offer and become your newest email subscriber!

But where will people see your free content?

### Promotion

You'll promote your valuable content in places where your ideal client already hangs out. This includes online places like social media, but also at events, workshops, interviews, sponsorships and through advertising. Promotion is the way new potential customers find out about you. From there, they read your free content and then become email subscribers. So when do you make sales?

### Nurture and Convert

Sales come from your email list, but you have to be thoughtful. You can't just make sales offers every day to your email list. Instead, you want to "nurture" your new subscriber by sending useful emails that continue to build your relationship and establish credibility, and then make occasional relevant offers. When an email subscriber buys one of your offers, that's called a "conversion" — she's just become a paying customer! And of course, she stays part of your email list so you can continue to build your relationship and make more offers over time.

Before moving on to the next step in the planner, talk yourself through the Organic Growth System diagram from left to right. Can you see the path for how a website visitor becomes a paying client? Can you see how building this type of relationship is just like any personal relationship you have? You increasingly build trust and engagement before she's ready to buy from you. And following this system makes it easy and natural to do that!

Now that you understand the flow from initial interaction to paying client, let's map out the Organic Growth System for your business.

You may have some or all of this system set up already. Just fill in as much as you know now. You can add to this page as you work through the remainder of the planner, where we'll go into each step in greater detail.

## Wellpreneur Organic Growth System

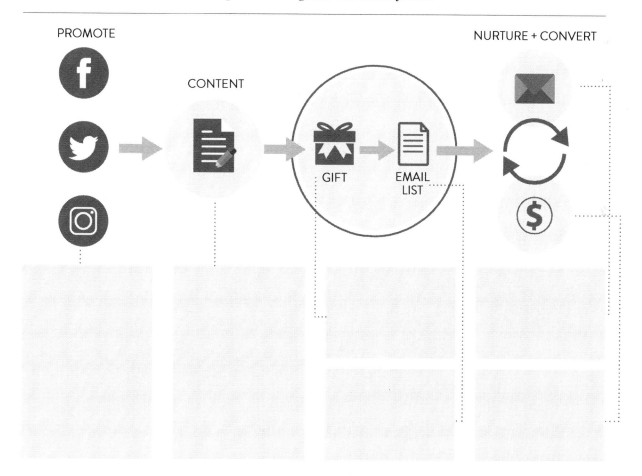

Which steps in the Organic Growth System do you need to create?

As you think through the flow from initial interaction to client,
are there any holes, gaps or areas that don't make sense?

Before we look at each step of your Organic Growth System in detail, we need to reconnect with your ideal client. Your entire marketing approach depends on WHO you're trying to reach. If your ideal customer is a 32 year old stay-at-home mom, you're going to approach her very differently than a 50 year old male corporate executive. You'd use different language, social media platforms and offers. So first let's reconnect with YOUR ideal customer, and then we'll build out the system to reach her.

## YOUR IDEAL CLIENT

The success of your products, services and marketing relies on how well you know your ideal customer. I like to do this by describing the situation of *one* ideal customer. Your marketing is more effective if you write specifically to one person, so let's get to know her here. If you know a real person who is your ideal client, you can describe her here, otherwise just imagine someone. You may want to find a picture of a person in a magazine who represents your ideal client and include it here.

Name:

Age:

Where does she live?

Does she work? Where?

What is the major problem you solve for your customer? Be specific.

What was her life like before working with you?
What were her pain points and frustrations?

What are her big questions and fears?

What are her dreams?

List 10 places where your ideal customer hangs out online or goes to for information and advice. Be specific. This could be websites, social media groups, hashtags she uses, influencers she follows or blogs she reads.

1. _____
2. _____
3. _____
4. _____
5. _____
6. _____
7. _____
8. _____
9. _____
10. _____

# IDEAL CLIENT ACTION STEPS

///////////

*Write any tasks or to-dos that came up during the ideal client exercise here.*

- ○ _____
- ○ _____
- ○ _____
- ○ _____
- ○ _____
- ○ _____
- ○ _____
- ○ _____
- ○ _____
- ○ _____
- ○ _____
- ○ _____
- ○ _____
- ○ _____

# PRODUCTS AND SERVICES

Now that you know WHO your ideal customer is, let's look at what you'll sell her. Another way to say it is, how will you generate revenue in your business this year?

List the products and services you currently sell and how much revenue they generated in the last 12 months. We listed last year's revenue earlier in the planner, but this breaks it down so we see where the revenue came from! Don't forget to list out all the ways your business received money, including revenue from coaching, ebooks, affiliate and referral commissions, network marketing, selling physical products and any other income . If it brought in revenue, include it below!

| PRODUCT/SERVICE | PRICE | # SOLD IN LAST YEAR | $ REVENUE |
|---|---|---|---|
|  |  |  |  |
|  |  |  |  |
|  |  |  |  |
|  |  |  |  |
|  |  |  |  |
|  |  |  |  |
|  |  |  |  |
|  |  |  |  |

Now let's look at your vision of the future. What products are you dreaming about creating? *(Refer back to the Big Dream section of this planner).*

How much money do you want your business to make this year? Be specific.

How will you reach your revenue goal?
It's easier to manage on a monthly basis,
so just divide your annual goal by 12 and write it here:

Next, for each of your products (current and future), how many of each would you need to sell to reach your monthly goal? For example, if you want to make $10,000 per month, you could sell 10 products or services that cost $1,000 each, or 100 products or services that cost $100 each, or more likely, some combination of products and services at various price points. You might write down a few different scenarios to reach your revenue goal and then see which scenario feels the best. Again, don't forget to include ALL the ways your business receives revenue. Make sure to include existing products that you want to keep, plus the new products you're dreaming about creating.

| PRODUCT/SERVICE | PRICE | $ REVENUE |
|---|---|---|
| | | |
| | | |
| | | |
| | | |
| | | |
| | | |
| | | |
| | | |

# PRODUCTS AND SERVICES ACTION STEPS

//////////

*Record any action steps or to-dos from the product planning section here.*

○ _____

○ _____

○ _____

○ _____

○ _____

○ _____

○ _____

○ _____

○ _____

○ _____

○ _____

○ _____

○ _____

○ _____

○ _____

Now you know what you're going to sell this year and to who. Let's turn our focus now to your valuable free content.

Consistently creating valuable free content attracts potential clients to your business and establishes you as an expert who can help solve their problems. This is the basis of the Organic Growth System.

There are two secrets for successful content:
1.  Creating what your ideal client wants to consume, not simply what you want to create.
2.  Consistency.

**What kind of content are you going to produce?**
Content falls into 3 categories: written (blogs), audio (podcasts) and video. I suggest you focus on one type of content. Choose what you're good at producing (what seems fun and easy?), and consider what your ideal client likes to consume (does she love or hate online video?).

Commit to the type of content you're going to create. Write it here:

**Frequency**

How often will you produce content? Don't overcommit yourself here. Somewhere between weekly and monthly is probably right. Some people produce daily content but think long and hard about that before you commit to it — content creation is a marathon!

I've found it's more effective to create content less regularly, but then promote it more (ie, share it more on social media or with other bloggers or media outlets) than creating a lot of content and not having time or resources to promote it.

How often will you release new content?

**How much will you need?**

Based on the frequency you chose above, how much content will you need to produce this year? If you chose weekly content, then you'll need 52 pieces of content during the year. Monthly content? You'll need 12 pieces of content for the year.

How many pieces will you need to create?

**The Secret to Easy Content Creation**

As I said before, creating content is a marathon. But you can make it easier. The best way I've found to be consistent with content is to create an editorial calendar. Your editorial calendar tells you exactly what you're going to publish and when, so you never get stuck wondering what to write about! I'll walk you through the process.

STEP 1: FREE FLOW BRAINSTORMING.

Set a timer for 10 minutes. On the next page, write down potential content ideas (ie, blog post titles, podcast episodes, video topics etc.). Don't censor yourself, just brainstorm. Here are some questions to ask yourself:

- What am I really excited to write about?
- What are the top questions (FAQ's) that people ask me about my subject area?
- What is trendy or topical in my industry right now?
- What are the top mistakes that people make in my subject area?
- What do people THINK is good for them in my subject area, but really isn't?
- What do I wish I could go back and tell myself when I was a beginner?
- What are my top 5 tips for people in my subject area?
- What are my top recommended resources (websites, books etc.) in my subject area?

## STEP 2: WALK AWAY FROM THE LIST FOR A FEW MINUTES TO CLEAR YOUR HEAD.

Now review what you wrote about your ideal client earlier in the workbook and then read through your content ideas, putting a star beside those which most answer your client's questions or solve her big problems.

## STEP 3: HOW MANY IDEAS ARE STARRED?

Review the list again, and pick out your top 10 ideas. You'll create these first.

1. _____

2. _____

3. _____

4. _____

5. _____

6. _____

7. _____

8. _____

9. _____

10. _____

# EDITORIAL CALENDAR

You're almost there! Now you've got at least ten juicy content ideas, and the final step is to organize them into an editorial calendar so you know exactly what to create each week! Start the calendar this month and work outwards for the coming year. Begin with the top 10 topics from Step 3 and then add more to complete the calendar.

I've included space below to plan your entire year, but I often plan only six months of content at a time, so it feels fresh and current (and so I can adjust topics based on what's working.) Follow the frequency you set earlier, so if you're releasing content monthly, only list one piece of content per month. If it's weekly, you'll need four pieces of content per month. Feel free to add in a few breaks for holidays or life events in the coming year. Remember there's a detailed monthly planning section at the end of this planner, so you can schedule each piece of content on a calendar.

| MONTH 1 | |
|---|---|
| DATE | TOPIC |
|  |  |
|  |  |
|  |  |
|  |  |

| MONTH 2 | |
|---|---|
| DATE | TOPIC |
|  |  |
|  |  |
|  |  |
|  |  |

| MONTH 3 | |
|---|---|
| DATE | TOPIC |
|  |  |
|  |  |
|  |  |
|  |  |

| MONTH 4 | |
|---|---|
| DATE | TOPIC |
| | |
| | |
| | |

| MONTH 5 | |
|---|---|
| DATE | TOPIC |
| | |
| | |
| | |

| MONTH 6 | |
|---|---|
| DATE | TOPIC |
| | |
| | |
| | |

| MONTH 7 | |
|---|---|
| DATE | TOPIC |
| | |
| | |
| | |

| MONTH 8 | |
|---|---|
| DATE | TOPIC |
| | |
| | |
| | |

| MONTH 9 | |
|---|---|
| DATE | TOPIC |
| | |
| | |
| | |

| MONTH 10 | |
|---|---|
| DATE | TOPIC |
| | |
| | |
| | |
| | |

| MONTH 11 | |
|---|---|
| DATE | TOPIC |
| | |
| | |
| | |
| | |

| MONTH 12 | |
|---|---|
| DATE | TOPIC |
| | |
| | |
| | |
| | |

# CONTENT ACTION STEPS

//////////

*Record any action steps or to-dos from the content planning section here.*

- ○ _____
- ○ _____
- ○ _____
- ○ _____
- ○ _____
- ○ _____
- ○ _____
- ○ _____
- ○ _____
- ○ _____
- ○ _____
- ○ _____
- ○ _____
- ○ _____
- ○ _____
- ○ _____

# ALL ABOUT EMAIL

Let's see where we are so far. We know your ideal client and the products/services you'll sell. You've also created an editorial calendar of valuable content that will interest your ideal client. Now let's shift our focus to building your relationship. Remember, there are two parts: getting the right people onto your list and keeping in touch with your subscribers.

## Opt-In Gift

Think about what you're currently offering your clients.

What happens once they find your content? What is their next step?

What is your email opt-in gift?

How is it delivered?

What should the potential client do next after viewing your gift?
What is the Call to Action?

How could you change your current email opt-in gift to attract more people?

What kind of support will you need to make these changes?

**Nurturing**

Do you send a regular email newsletter or an automated email sequence (autoresponder)?

How often do your email subscribers hear from you?

What's included in your email newsletter?

How could you change your current approach to build a stronger relationship with your customers?

What kind of support will you need to make these changes?

# EMAIL ACTION STEPS

//////////

*Capture any action items or to-dos from the email section here.*

○ _____

○ _____

○ _____

○ _____

○ _____

○ _____

○ _____

○ _____

○ _____

○ _____

○ _____

○ _____

○ _____

○ _____

○ _____

○ _____

# PROMOTION

Once you've gotten your editorial calendar sorted and you know how you'll work to improve your opt-in offer, you can focus on how you're going to get more eyes on your free content. Remember, the goal is for potential customers to find your free content so valuable they'll sign up for your email list to continue to learn from you.

A common mistake is to create content, share it on social media one time, and then never mention it again! If you're creating relevant content, you'll want to promote it over and over again because while your existing audience may have seen it, none of your new ideal clients will have, and it's still valuable for them! So you'll want to keep promoting both your new and old content as you go.

The key with promotion is that you need to promote *where your ideal customer already hangs out online*. So, choose your platforms wisely. You can't be everywhere, but you do need to consistently promote your content in the right places.

Where does your ideal customer hang out online? You might refer back to the list you created for your ideal client earlier. Think of social media sites, blogs, forums, podcasts, YouTube, online magazines, and any other relevant option.

What are your top 2 promotional  platforms? Choose the 2 from the list above that you'll be able to promote to regularly and which seem fun and easy to you.

For each focus platform, let's dig into how you'll use it.

## PLATFORM 1:

### What kind of content will you promote on this platform?

### How often will you promote on this platform?

### What will you need to create to promote there effectively? For example, do you need to write a short promotional blurb or create an engaging image? How are other people successfully using this platform? What has worked for you in the past?

### What resources, support or tools will you need to be successful on that platform?

**PLATFORM 2:**

What kind of content will you promote on this platform?

How often will you promote on this platform?

What will you need to create to promote there effectively? For example, do you need to write a short promotional blurb or create an engaging image? How are other people successfully using this platform? What has worked for you in the past?

What resources, support or tools will you need to be successful on that platform?

# PROMOTION ACTION STEPS

////////////

*Record any action steps or to-dos from the promotion section here.*

- ○ _____
- ○ _____
- ○ _____
- ○ _____
- ○ _____
- ○ _____
- ○ _____
- ○ _____
- ○ _____
- ○ _____
- ○ _____
- ○ _____
- ○ _____
- ○ _____
- ○ _____
- ○ _____

## PRIORITIES

You've just filled this planner with big dreams, plans and lots of action steps to create your ideal business and life. You may be excited to get started, or you might be feeling overwhelmed at everything that needs to be done!

It's amazing how much you can accomplish in a year, if you just take it one step at a time.

In this section, we're going to compile all your action steps, and prioritize them, so you know where to start.

List out the action steps you've identified throughout the planner. You'll want to look back at the Organic Growth System as well as the checklists at the end of each section. Write your action items in the appropriate section below:

| YOUR IDEAL CLIENT | EMAIL |
|---|---|
| | |
| | |
| | |
| | |
| | |

## CONTENT

## PROMOTION

## PRODUCTS AND SERVICES

## OTHER

Great! Now you might have noticed I shuffled around the order of the sections in the list above. That's because I've put them in order of priority for setting up a sustainable online business. Here are my recommended priorities (for online marketing) in more detail. You might go back and adjust your action items as you read through this list. Once you've completed a step, just cross it off the list.

- ○ Identify a specific ideal client for your business.
- ○ Set up an email list using an email marketing service.
- ○ Create an awesome opt-in offer (and put it on your website or landing page).
- ○ Set your editorial calendar and begin creating content.
- ○ Promote your content and your opt-in to gain subscribers.

  *Note: You can do all of the above, even if you haven't started a business yet — it's never too early to build an audience!*

- ○ Create a product or service.
- ○ Set up an automatic email sequence to introduce the product to your subscribers.
- ○ Get your product/service in the hands of customers, get feedback and improve it.
- ○ Create and launch additional products and services.

Feel free to adjust action items based on your own priorities and business goals. But if you feel stuck, use my recommended priorities to guide where you'll start this year.

Next, we'll spread these action items out across the next 12 months, so you have time to make them happen!

With your list of priorities in hand, let's explore the rhythm of your year, month by month, so you can bring your big vision into being. This is where we break down that list above into smaller parts that you can work on each month. This section gives you a feel for the flow of your year, so you know when you're going to have a period of intense work, a product launch, a vacation, a sale, etc. Remember, there's a detailed monthly planning section at the end of this planner, so you can expand on each month's actions. For now, just include the broad strokes, not every little action item.

For each month, you'll want to include:

- Target monthly revenue (from the products/services section)
- Promotional focus. Is there a specific focus that month such as a new product launch, event, sale, holiday, etc?
- Setting up your Organic Growth System. These are the prioritized action steps from the previous system. Start at the top of the list and plan to complete one or two per month this year.
- Major projects. These are the other big projects which came up in the dreaming section of the planner. You may or may not have these. Examples might include creating a new online program, writing a book, starting a podcast, etc.
- Personal life events and vacations! Take your personal life obligations into account when planning out your year.

## MONTH 1

TARGET REVENUE

PROMOTIONAL FOCUS

ORGANIC GROWTH
SYSTEM FOCUS

MAJOR PROJECTS

PERSONAL

OTHER

## MONTH 2

TARGET REVENUE

PROMOTIONAL FOCUS

ORGANIC GROWTH
SYSTEM FOCUS

MAJOR PROJECTS

PERSONAL

OTHER

# MONTH 3

TARGET REVENUE

PROMOTIONAL FOCUS

ORGANIC GROWTH
SYSTEM FOCUS

MAJOR PROJECTS

PERSONAL

OTHER

# MONTH 4

TARGET REVENUE

PROMOTIONAL FOCUS

ORGANIC GROWTH
SYSTEM FOCUS

MAJOR PROJECTS

PERSONAL

OTHER

# MONTH 5

TARGET REVENUE

PROMOTIONAL FOCUS

ORGANIC GROWTH
SYSTEM FOCUS

MAJOR PROJECTS

PERSONAL

OTHER

## MONTH 6

TARGET REVENUE

PROMOTIONAL FOCUS

ORGANIC GROWTH
SYSTEM FOCUS

MAJOR PROJECTS

PERSONAL

OTHER

# MONTH 7

TARGET REVENUE

PROMOTIONAL FOCUS

ORGANIC GROWTH
SYSTEM FOCUS

MAJOR PROJECTS

PERSONAL

OTHER

# MONTH 8

TARGET REVENUE

PROMOTIONAL FOCUS

ORGANIC GROWTH
SYSTEM FOCUS

MAJOR PROJECTS

PERSONAL

OTHER

# MONTH 9

TARGET REVENUE

PROMOTIONAL FOCUS

ORGANIC GROWTH
SYSTEM FOCUS

MAJOR PROJECTS

PERSONAL

OTHER

# MONTH 10

TARGET REVENUE

PROMOTIONAL FOCUS

ORGANIC GROWTH
SYSTEM FOCUS

MAJOR PROJECTS

PERSONAL

OTHER

# MONTH 11

TARGET REVENUE

PROMOTIONAL FOCUS

ORGANIC GROWTH
SYSTEM FOCUS

MAJOR PROJECTS

PERSONAL

OTHER

# MONTH 12

TARGET REVENUE

PROMOTIONAL FOCUS

ORGANIC GROWTH
SYSTEM FOCUS

MAJOR PROJECTS

PERSONAL

OTHER

Almost there!

At this point in the planner, you'll:

- See a clear vision for your life and business this year.
- Understand how new clients will discover your business, join your email list and become paying clients.
- Have a prioritized list of tasks to grow your business through online marketing.
- Feel how the tasks will spread out across the year.

Now that you have your plan for the year, we're going to look at the schedule, habits and support needed to take consistent action.

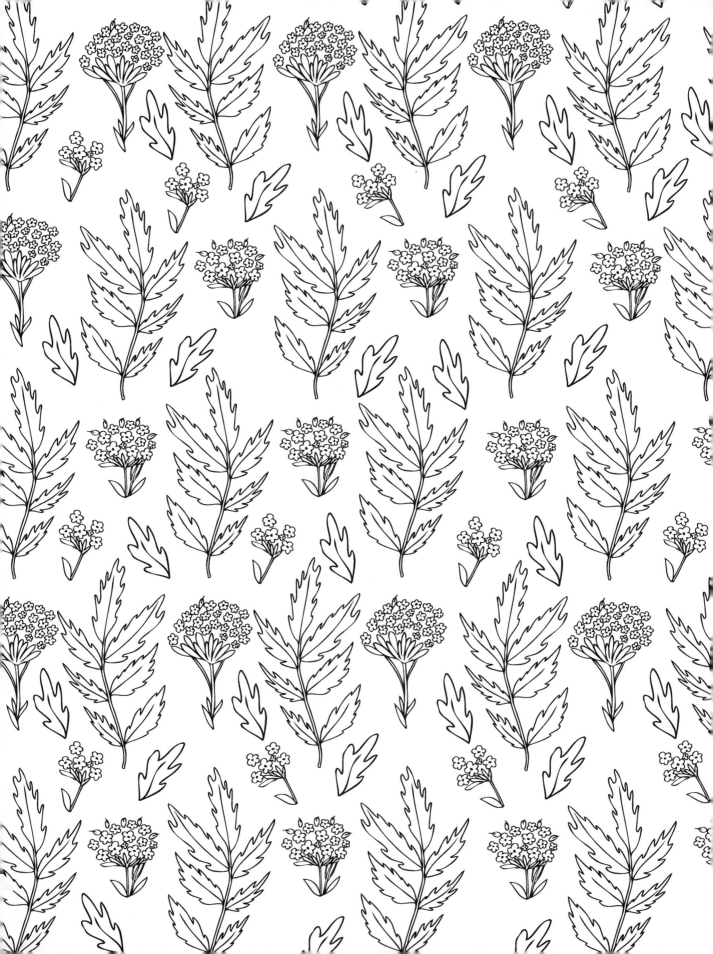

# MAKING
# IT
# HAPPEN

---

## YOUR WEEKLY SCHEDULE

As a wellpreneur, you know the easiest way to adopt a new healthy habit is to make it routine so you don't have to think about it. I've found it's similar in business. There are certain activities that need to happen regularly to keep your business running and your audience growing. If you can automate these tasks, you can focus your precious creative energy on the big projects, like creating new products, preparing a talk or writing that book!

I know that as creative business owners seeking freedom and flexibility, we can be a bit resistant to having a schedule. But I'd like to encourage you to try blocking chunks of time to handle the recurring tasks in your business. It's less stressful and it actually gives you MORE time for the fun, creative work that you love. Personally, I find hourly scheduling too restrictive, so I like to block in half days (mornings / afternoons).

If you have a day job, limited childcare, or other daily commitments, you could use different blocks of time, for example, before work, lunch break, evening or perhaps half-day blocks on the weekends. Time blocking your schedule is totally unique to you. What fits your needs?

Here are the tasks you'll want to schedule each week (adjust to fit your business):

- Working with clients
- Creating content
- Publishing content (this can often be scheduled in advance)
- Promotional activities including scheduling posts on social media
- Engaging with your audience on social media
- Self-care and exercise
- Major projects (like creating a new product or preparing a talk)
- Admin (accounting, website plugin updates, etc.)

Remember: You don't need to create the 'perfect' schedule. Simply assign blocks of time that feel realistic for you. Try your new schedule for a week or two and then review and adjust so it fits your life.

You can create your weekly time-blocked schedule on the next page. Feel free to change the blocks of time to fit your life.

|  | EARLY MORNING | MORNING | LUNCH | EARLY AFTERNOON | LATE AFTERNOON | DINNER | EVENING |
|---|---|---|---|---|---|---|---|
| MONDAY | | | | | | | |
| TUESDAY | | | | | | | |
| WEDNESDAY | | | | | | | |
| THURSDAY | | | | | | | |
| FRIDAY | | | | | | | |
| SATURDAY | | | | | | | |
| SUNDAY | | | | | | | |

# SUPPORT

Looking at what you want to accomplish this year, what support will you need? Let yourself open to the possibility of support, which can come in paid and unpaid forms. Consider where you could use more support in each area and write it below. You're not committing to it yet — you're just opening yourself up to the possibility.

Peers/masterminds:

High-level coaching/education:

Business task support (virtual assistant, designer, website developer, etc.):

Family/household support
*(asking family members to take on more tasks, cleaning service, grocery delivery, etc.):*

Personal support (trainer, assistant, delivery service etc.):

Even with your best intentions to have a balanced, joyful, flowing life and business, stress, worry, deadlines and frustration will happen. This page is for those times. A little thought right now about how to get yourself out of a funk will be a lifesaver in those moments when you don't have the perspective to shift your frame of mind!

What are some simple things you can do when you feel discouraged, frustrated or sad that will help you feel better? For example, exercise, sunshine, baths, dark chocolate, calling a friend, or anything else you find relaxing or that makes you feel good.

On the next page, write an 'open in case of emergency' letter to yourself for that moment when you're frustrated, fed up and want to quit!

# OPEN IN CASE OF EMERGENCY...

This is a fun one if it appeals to you. It taps into your inner wisdom and knowing. Take a few minutes to close your eyes and get centered. Imagine you're going to meet Future You — yourself in 10 years. See yourself opening the door and walking into the room where your future self is. What does she look like? Where is she? What does she say to you? In what ways can she encourage you? What advice does she have? Feel into this vision for a few minutes, then open your eyes and write a letter from Future You to yourself today.

DATE (10 years in the future):

Dear

# A PLEDGE

I am wholeheartedly open to the potential and possibilities of the next twelve months.

I promise to show up with my best self and take action to move
my business and life forward, even in a small way, every day.

I promise to take care of myself as I grow my business and will
schedule time to take care of me, every week.

I know that I can always expand to a new level of abundance and joy.

I believe that abundance and joy are infinite, and that by increasing mine,
there is also more than enough for everyone else so that we can all rise together

*Add your own commitments here...*

_____

_____

_____

_____

I am open to the synchronicities, possibilities and wonder of this year. And so it is.

Signed: _____     Date: _____

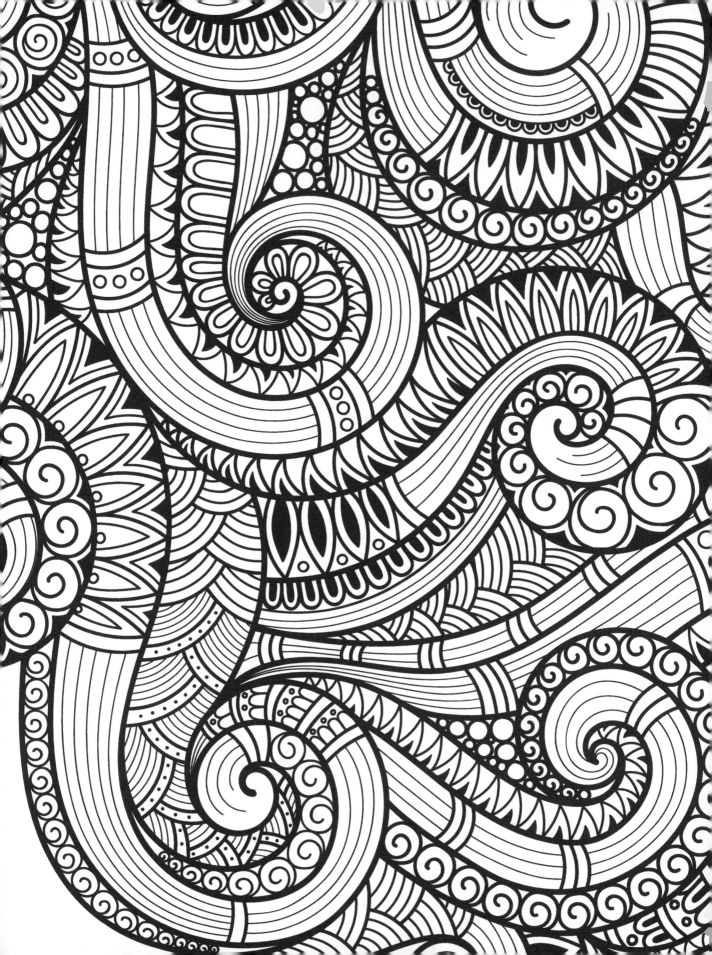

# MONTHLY PLANNING & RESULTS

/////////////

This section of the planner is your monthly planning and progress tracker. Use it to plan each month and track your results and growth stats.

Each month has four planner pages. There's space to include the tasks and focus areas from your Month by Month planning, as well as a blank calendar to plan your work. You'll use the monthly review page at the end of each month to record your results. There are two blank pages per month for additional brainstorming, action items, writing or plans.

Get ready to be amazed at your progress!

## MONTH

| MONDAY | TUESDAY | WEDNESDAY | THURSDAY | FRIDAY | SATURDAY | SUNDAY |
|--------|---------|-----------|----------|--------|----------|--------|
|        |         |           |          |        |          |        |
|        |         |           |          |        |          |        |
|        |         |           |          |        |          |        |
|        |         |           |          |        |          |        |
|        |         |           |          |        |          |        |

### REVENUE GOAL

### PROMOTIONAL FOCUS

### KEY ACTIONS

○ _____    ○ _____

○ _____    ○ _____

○ _____    ○ _____

○ _____    ○ _____

## END OF MONTH METRICS

Revenue

# Email Subscribers

Social Media Followers

WINS

CHALLENGES

## LESSONS LEARNED

## MONTH

| MONDAY | TUESDAY | WEDNESDAY | THURSDAY | FRIDAY | SATURDAY | SUNDAY |
|--------|---------|-----------|----------|--------|----------|--------|
|        |         |           |          |        |          |        |
|        |         |           |          |        |          |        |
|        |         |           |          |        |          |        |
|        |         |           |          |        |          |        |
|        |         |           |          |        |          |        |

### REVENUE GOAL

### PROMOTIONAL FOCUS

### KEY ACTIONS

○ _____    ○ _____

○ _____    ○ _____

○ _____    ○ _____

○ _____    ○ _____

## END OF MONTH METRICS

Revenue

Social Media Followers

# Email Subscribers

WINS

CHALLENGES

LESSONS LEARNED

THE WELLPRENEUR PLANNER

## MONTH

| MONDAY | TUESDAY | WEDNESDAY | THURSDAY | FRIDAY | SATURDAY | SUNDAY |
|--------|---------|-----------|----------|--------|----------|--------|
|  |  |  |  |  |  |  |
|  |  |  |  |  |  |  |
|  |  |  |  |  |  |  |
|  |  |  |  |  |  |  |
|  |  |  |  |  |  |  |

### REVENUE GOAL

### PROMOTIONAL FOCUS

### KEY ACTIONS

- ⭕ _____
- ⭕ _____
- ⭕ _____
- ⭕ _____

- ⭕ _____
- ⭕ _____
- ⭕ _____
- ⭕ _____

## END OF MONTH METRICS

Revenue

Social Media Followers

# Email Subscribers

WINS

CHALLENGES

LESSONS LEARNED

# MONTH

| MONDAY | TUESDAY | WEDNESDAY | THURSDAY | FRIDAY | SATURDAY | SUNDAY |
|--------|---------|-----------|----------|--------|----------|--------|
|        |         |           |          |        |          |        |
|        |         |           |          |        |          |        |
|        |         |           |          |        |          |        |
|        |         |           |          |        |          |        |
|        |         |           |          |        |          |        |

## REVENUE GOAL

## PROMOTIONAL FOCUS

## KEY ACTIONS

- ◯ _____
- ◯ _____
- ◯ _____
- ◯ _____

- ◯ _____
- ◯ _____
- ◯ _____
- ◯ _____

## END OF MONTH METRICS

Revenue

Social Media Followers

# Email Subscribers

WINS

CHALLENGES

LESSONS LEARNED

# MONTH

| MONDAY | TUESDAY | WEDNESDAY | THURSDAY | FRIDAY | SATURDAY | SUNDAY |
|--------|---------|-----------|----------|--------|----------|--------|
|  |  |  |  |  |  |  |
|  |  |  |  |  |  |  |
|  |  |  |  |  |  |  |
|  |  |  |  |  |  |  |
|  |  |  |  |  |  |  |

## REVENUE GOAL

## PROMOTIONAL FOCUS

## KEY ACTIONS

○ _____    ○ _____

○ _____    ○ _____

○ _____    ○ _____

○ _____    ○ _____

## END OF MONTH METRICS

Revenue

Social Media Followers

# Email Subscribers

WINS

CHALLENGES

## LESSONS LEARNED

# MONTH

| MONDAY | TUESDAY | WEDNESDAY | THURSDAY | FRIDAY | SATURDAY | SUNDAY |
|---|---|---|---|---|---|---|
| | | | | | | |
| | | | | | | |
| | | | | | | |
| | | | | | | |
| | | | | | | |

### REVENUE GOAL

### PROMOTIONAL FOCUS

### KEY ACTIONS

○ _____     ○ _____

○ _____     ○ _____

○ _____     ○ _____

○ _____     ○ _____

END OF MONTH METRICS

Revenue

Social Media Followers

# Email Subscribers

WINS

CHALLENGES

LESSONS LEARNED

## MONTH

| MONDAY | TUESDAY | WEDNESDAY | THURSDAY | FRIDAY | SATURDAY | SUNDAY |
|--------|---------|-----------|----------|--------|----------|--------|
|        |         |           |          |        |          |        |
|        |         |           |          |        |          |        |
|        |         |           |          |        |          |        |
|        |         |           |          |        |          |        |
|        |         |           |          |        |          |        |

### REVENUE GOAL

### PROMOTIONAL FOCUS

### KEY ACTIONS

○ _____    ○ _____

○ _____    ○ _____

○ _____    ○ _____

○ _____    ○ _____

## END OF MONTH METRICS

Revenue

Social Media Followers

# Email Subscribers

WINS

CHALLENGES

LESSONS LEARNED

# MONTH

| MONDAY | TUESDAY | WEDNESDAY | THURSDAY | FRIDAY | SATURDAY | SUNDAY |
|--------|---------|-----------|----------|--------|----------|--------|
|        |         |           |          |        |          |        |
|        |         |           |          |        |          |        |
|        |         |           |          |        |          |        |
|        |         |           |          |        |          |        |
|        |         |           |          |        |          |        |

## REVENUE GOAL

## PROMOTIONAL FOCUS

## KEY ACTIONS

- ○ _____
- ○ _____
- ○ _____
- ○ _____

- ○ _____
- ○ _____
- ○ _____
- ○ _____

END OF MONTH METRICS

Revenue

Social Media Followers

# Email Subscribers

WINS

CHALLENGES

LESSONS LEARNED

## MONTH

| MONDAY | TUESDAY | WEDNESDAY | THURSDAY | FRIDAY | SATURDAY | SUNDAY |
|--------|---------|-----------|----------|--------|----------|--------|
|        |         |           |          |        |          |        |
|        |         |           |          |        |          |        |
|        |         |           |          |        |          |        |
|        |         |           |          |        |          |        |
|        |         |           |          |        |          |        |

### REVENUE GOAL

### PROMOTIONAL FOCUS

### KEY ACTIONS

○ _____    ○ _____

○ _____    ○ _____

○ _____    ○ _____

○ _____    ○ _____

END OF MONTH METRICS

Revenue

# Email Subscribers

Social Media Followers

WINS

CHALLENGES

LESSONS LEARNED

## MONTH

| MONDAY | TUESDAY | WEDNESDAY | THURSDAY | FRIDAY | SATURDAY | SUNDAY |
|---|---|---|---|---|---|---|
|  |  |  |  |  |  |  |
|  |  |  |  |  |  |  |
|  |  |  |  |  |  |  |
|  |  |  |  |  |  |  |
|  |  |  |  |  |  |  |

### REVENUE GOAL

### PROMOTIONAL FOCUS

### KEY ACTIONS

- ○ _____
- ○ _____
- ○ _____
- ○ _____

- ○ _____
- ○ _____
- ○ _____
- ○ _____

## END OF MONTH METRICS

Revenue

Social Media Followers

# Email Subscribers

WINS

CHALLENGES

LESSONS LEARNED

## MONTH

| MONDAY | TUESDAY | WEDNESDAY | THURSDAY | FRIDAY | SATURDAY | SUNDAY |
|--------|---------|-----------|----------|--------|----------|--------|
|        |         |           |          |        |          |        |
|        |         |           |          |        |          |        |
|        |         |           |          |        |          |        |
|        |         |           |          |        |          |        |
|        |         |           |          |        |          |        |

### REVENUE GOAL

### PROMOTIONAL FOCUS

### KEY ACTIONS

- ○ _____
- ○ _____
- ○ _____
- ○ _____

- ○ _____
- ○ _____
- ○ _____
- ○ _____

## END OF MONTH METRICS

Revenue

Social Media Followers

# Email Subscribers

WINS

CHALLENGES

LESSONS LEARNED

# MONTH

| MONDAY | TUESDAY | WEDNESDAY | THURSDAY | FRIDAY | SATURDAY | SUNDAY |
|--------|---------|-----------|----------|--------|----------|--------|
|        |         |           |          |        |          |        |
|        |         |           |          |        |          |        |
|        |         |           |          |        |          |        |
|        |         |           |          |        |          |        |
|        |         |           |          |        |          |        |

## REVENUE GOAL

## PROMOTIONAL FOCUS

## KEY ACTIONS

◯ _____    ◯ _____

◯ _____    ◯ _____

◯ _____    ◯ _____

◯ _____    ◯ _____

END OF MONTH METRICS

Revenue

Social Media Followers

# Email Subscribers

WINS

CHALLENGES

LESSONS LEARNED

THE WELLPRENEUR PLANNER

# Congratulations!

You just finished a remarkable and wisdom-filled year in your life and business. Take a moment to appreciate your incredible personal and business growth.

Now it's time to continue your cycle of growth and plan the next 12 months. Get a fresh copy of this planner to review last year and plan the next! Or simply go through the last year review section again to see how far you've come.

But first, let us celebrate this year with you! Share a picture with the wellpreneur community using the hashtag #wellpreneurplanner. I'd love to see what you've created!

Dream big and keep going!

Amanda

*Wellpreneur: The Ultimate Guide for Wellness Entrepreneurs to Nail Your Niche and Find Clients Online.*

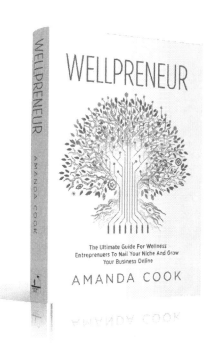

Why do some wellness entrepreneurs find freedom, flexibility and a healthy income online — while others get stuck spinning their wheels, never finding clients or making sales? It's not about who has the best website or who spends more time on social media. The secret is in the system.

Wellpreneurs who find clients online have a system in place that others don't. This system brings more of the right people to your website and turns them into paying clients. It's this proven, step-by-step system you'll learn in this book.

Wellpreneur is a guide to nailing your niche and finding more clients online, written just for wellness entrepreneurs. In the book you'll:

- Get total clarity on your target market, so you know exactly who you're serving (and why).
- Learn the proven five-step Organic Growth System to attract ideal prospects to your website and turn them into paying clients.
- Peek inside the businesses of successful wellpreneurs to learn how they grew  profitable wellness businesses online.
- Streamline your online marketing so you can spend less time marketing and more time doing work you love!

Available on Amazon. Download a free chapter at WellpreneurBook.com.

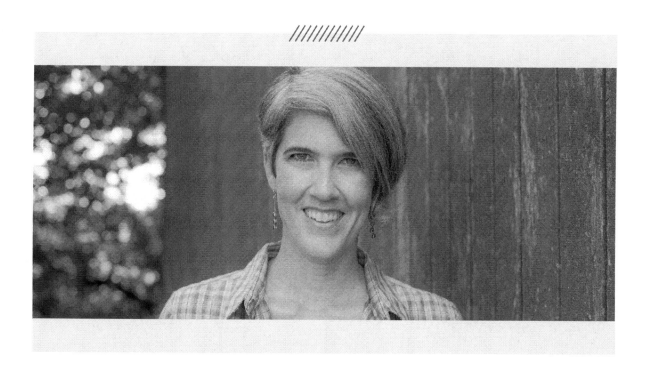

Amanda Cook is a digital storyteller, herbalist, host of The Wellpreneur Podcast and author of the bestselling book *Wellpreneur*. Her work has appeared in *The Huffington Post, The Sunday Telegraph, Natural Health Magazine, MindBodyGreen, TinyBuddha,* and *Copyblogger*. Originally from New Hampshire, Amanda currently lives in London, UK where she forages for wild plants along the Thames.

Discover more about Amanda's work at https://AmandaCook.me.

Connect with her on Instagram @AmandaCook.me

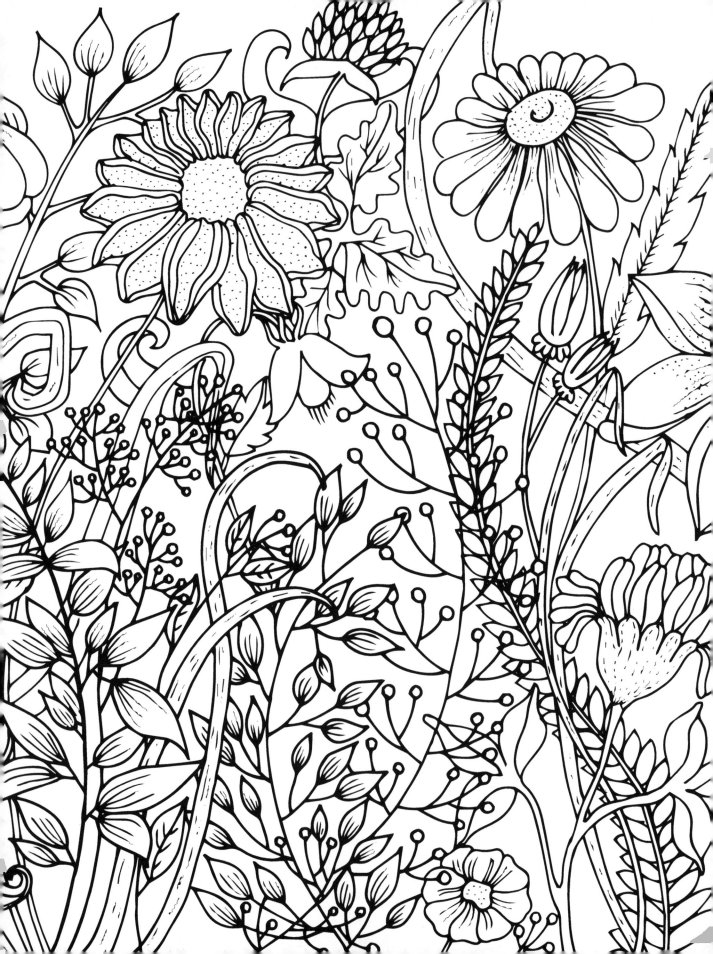

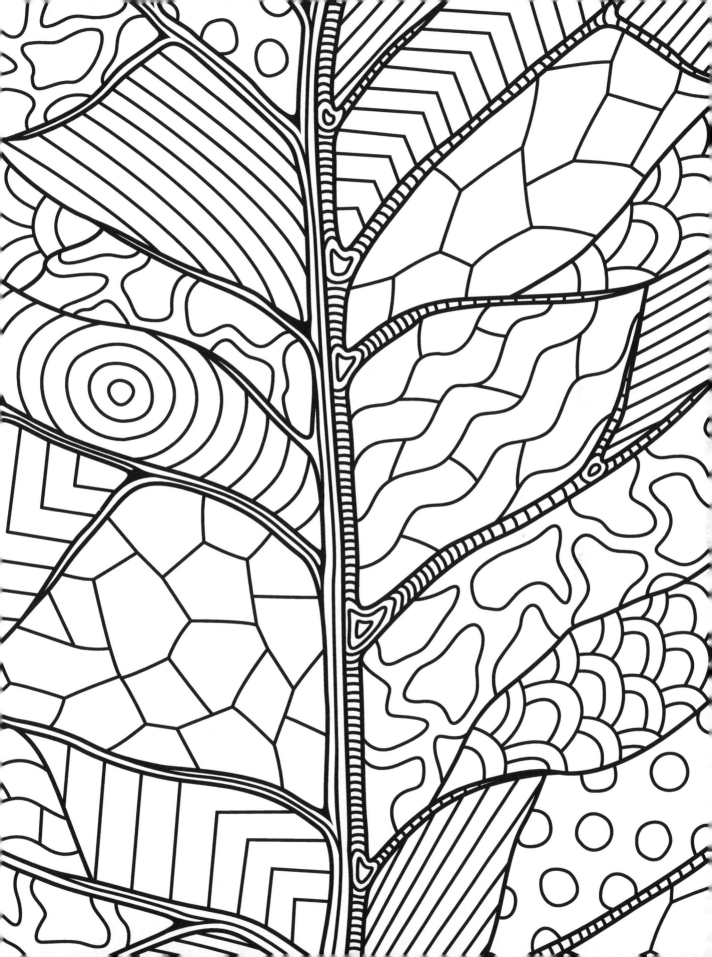

Made in the USA
Lexington, KY
27 November 2018